CLINICAL INTEGRATION

Accountable Care and Population Health

Third Edition [IN PRESS]

Chapter 11. Non-Traditional Mental Health and Substance Use Disorder Services as a Core Part of Health in CINs and ACOs

by

Roger Kathol, MD, DFAPA, FACP, CPE |
Susan Sargent, MBA | Steve Melek, FAAA |
Lee Sacks, MD | Kavita K. Patel MD, MS

BOOK EXECUTIVE EDITORS

Ken Yale | Thomas Raskauskas | J.M. Bohn | Colin Konschak

CONVURGENT
PUBLISHING

Convurgent Publishing, LLC
4445 Corporation Lane, Suite #227
Virginia Beach, VA 23462
Phone: (877) 254-9794, Fax: (757) 213-6801
Web Site: www.convurgent.com
E-mail: info@convurgent.com

Special Orders.
Bulk Quantity Sales.
Special discounts are available on quantity purchases. Please contact sales@convurgent.com.
Library of Congress Control Number: 2014953621
Bibliographic data:

Chapter 11. Non-Traditional Mental Health and Substance Use Disorder Services as a Core Part of Health in CINs and ACOs Clinical Integration, In: Accountable Care and Population Health, Third Edition. Chapter 11 Authors: Roger Kathol, Susan Sargent, Steve Melek, Lee Sacks, and Kavita K. Patel.

p. cm.
1. Clinical integration. 2. Clinically integrated networks. 3. Healthcare reform. 4. Health information technology. 5. Clinical quality. 6. Care coordination. 7. Behavioral health. 8. Population health.
ISBN: 978-0-9912345-2-3

ABOUT THIS CHAPTER

This chapter manuscript represents a final draft chapter to be incorporated in the forthcoming 3rd Edition of, *Clinical Integration. Accountable Care and Population Health*. The final version of this chapter will be subject to final revisioning by its authors and editing and copyediting by the executive editors and the publisher.

ABOUT THE CHAPTER 11 AUTHORS

Roger G. Kathol, MD, CPE, is president of Cartesian Solutions, Inc., is a health care consultant who assists employers, government agencies, health plans, hospitals and clinics, and care management vendors develop integrated medical and behavioral health programs for patients with high cost health complexity. Dr. Kathol is board certified in internal medicine, psychiatry, and medical management with extensive experience gained during 22 years as a physician/teacher/researcher at the University of Iowa and 16 years as an international health complexity and integrated health solutions, which improve care quality, augment outcomes, and lower total health care and health-related costs. Clients include: general hospitals and clinics, accountable care organizations; general medical health plans; case management programs and vendors; and employers and government agencies. Dr. Kathol is an adjunct professor of internal medicine and psychiatry at the University of Minnesota and has published over 165 peer reviewed articles and 25 book chapters.

Steve Melek, FSA, MAAA, is principal and consulting actuary with the Denver Health practice of Milliman. Steve's areas of expertise include healthcare product development, management, and financial analyses. He has worked extensively in the behavioral healthcare specialty field. He has worked with many managed behavioral healthcare organizations, parity issues and cost analyses, mental health utilization and costs in primary care settings, psychotropic drug treatment patterns, and strategic behavioral healthcare system design. He has experience with plan design, pricing, capitation and risk analysis, provider reimbursement analysis and strategies, healthcare revenue distribution, and utilization management analysis. He has completed valuations and projections of healthcare businesses and product lines, profitability and experience analysis, reinsurance analysis, pricing model and strategy development, and actuarial liability determination.

Susan C. Sargent, MBA, is president of Sargent Healthcare Management Advisors, LLC. Ms. Sargent has provided strategic planning, marketing, operations, and management assistance to healthcare providers nationally for over 25 years with a focus on bringing best practice medicine to best practice program and facility design. As such, she has worked with acute care general hospitals, multi-hospital systems, academic medical centers, and specialized civil, forensic and veterans' behavioral health facilities, contributing currency and fluency in the treatment, management, and operational issues facing providers. Sargent HMA is registered with the Central Contractor Registry (CCR) as a small business and a woman-owned business, and is certified as a woman business enterprise (WBE) in Pennsylvania, Delaware, and Virginia.

Lee Sacks, MD, has served as Executive Vice President, Chief Medical Officer since 1997 and is responsible for health outcomes, safety, clinical transformation, information systems, risk management/insurance, research and medical education and clinical laboratory services at Advocate Health Care. He also serves as Chief Executive Officer of Advocate Physician Partners, the clinically integrated network with 4,500 physicians serving 610,000 attributable lives. Modern Health Care recognized APP as the nation's largest ACO in 2013 and 2014. He serves as Chair of the ACL lab operating committee, the joint venture that provides laboratory services to the Advocate and Aurora systems.

Kavita K. Patel, MD, MS, is is a Fellow and Managing Director in the Engelberg Center for Health Care Reform at the Brookings Institution where she leads research on delivery system reforms, healthcare cost, physician payment and healthcare workforce productivity. Dr. Patel is, in addition, a practicing primary care physician at Johns Hopkins Medicine and a clinical instructor at UCLA's Geffen School of Medicine. Dr. Patel was previously a Director of Policy for The White House under President Obama and a senior advisor to the late Senator Edward Kennedy. Her prior research in healthcare quality and community approaches to mental illness have earned national recognition and she has published numerous papers and book chapters on healthcare reform and health policy. She has testified before Congress several times and she is a frequent guest expert on CBS, NBC and MSNBC as well as serving on the editorial board of the journal *Health Affairs*.

TABLE OF CONTENTS

Chapter 11. Non-Traditional Mental Health and Substance Use Disorder Services as a Core Part of Health in CINs and ACOs

Roger Kathol, MD, DFAPA, FACP, CPE | Susan Sargent, MBA
Steve Melek, FSA, FAAA | Lee Sacks, MD | Kavita K. Patel MD, MS

"After you've done a thing the same way for two years, look it over carefully. After five years, look at it with suspicion. And after ten years, throw it away and start all over."

Alfred Edward Perlman
1902-1983
President, Penn Central Transportation Company

Chapter 11 Learning Objectives

✓ To understand the frequency and interaction of behavioral health (BH) with general medical conditions.

✓ To summarize the way that BH services are currently delivered.

✓ To clarify the effect of currently siloed behavioral health payment practices on care delivery and patient outcomes.

✓ To review the clinical and cost impact of untreated behavioral health conditions in the medical setting.

✓ To describe models of value-added non-traditional behavioral health services to consider when building a CIN or ACO.

✓ To discuss the opportunity cost of behavioral health exclusion / marginalization when setting up a CIN or ACO.

Introduction

Mental health (MH) and substance use disorders (SUD), hereafter referred to as "behavioral health" (BH) conditions, present as emotional, behavioral, or cognitive disturbances, which interfere with a person's ability to function optimally while symptoms are present. Over eighty percent of patients with BH conditions present only or primarily in the primary or specialty medical/surgical setting, hereafter called "medical" setting (Figure 11-1). (Regier et al., 1993; Reilly et al., 2012; P. S. Wang et al., 2006) Of these, sixty to seventy percent receive no treatment for their BH conditions.(Kessler et al., 2005; P. S. Wang et al., 2007; P. S. Wang, Demler, & Kessler, 2002; P. S. Wang, Lane, et al., 2005) Fewer than one in nine of those who do receive treatment in the medical setting are exposed to a BH intervention that would be expected to improve symptoms or return a person to productive, psychological health.(P. S. Wang et al., 2002; P. S. Wang, Lane, et al., 2005)

Figure 11-1. Most BH Patients are Seen in the Medical Setting

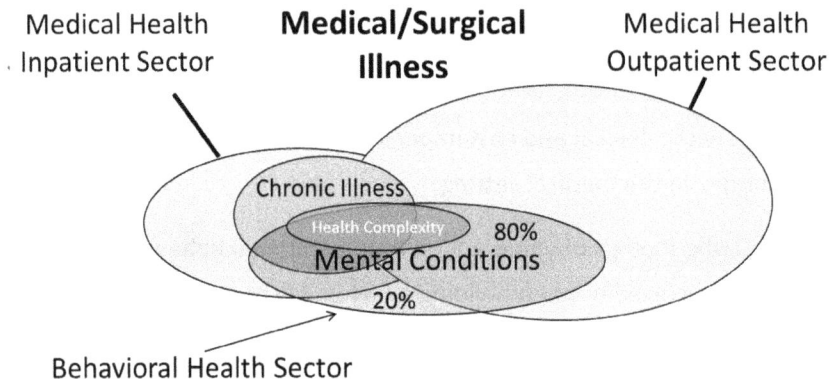

This Chapter will describe how BH services are delivered in today's health system; the influence that current payment practices have on how and where clinical services are delivered and where

BH professionals practice; the impact of isolated BH service delivery on the quality and cost of care within national, health plan, and clinic systems; the BH delivery system changes needed to improve health and cost outcomes of untreated BH conditions in the medical setting; and the opportunities associated with BH service implementation as a part of clinically integrated networks (CINs) and/or accountable care organizations (ACOs).

We posit that advanced CINs, such as those taking risk for total health and cost outcomes of populations of patients, including those developing ACOs, and many basic CINs that are providing integrated service delivery for targeted populations, will not meet basic Federal Trade Commission (FTC) or Department of Justice (DOJ) requirements inherent in CINs.(U.S. Department of Justice & Federal Trade Commission, 1996) That being, targeted improvement in quality and reducing cost through coordinated service delivery, unless they include "value-added" BH services and professionals as core CIN/ACO services and providers.

Today's BH Service Delivery

Over ninety-five percent of BH professionals practice almost exclusively in standalone inpatient (IP) and outpatient (OP) BH settings.(Franz et al., 2010) This is where the majority of evidence-based BH interventions are delivered.(P. S. Wang et al., 2007; P. S. Wang, Lane, et al., 2005) Specialty BH settings are designed to support treatment for patients with mild to serious BH conditions but especially cater to the delivery of services for those with serious and persistent primary BH disorders, such as schizophrenia, substance dependence, bipolar illness, serious eating disorders, autism, etc. Only fifteen to twenty percent of all patients with BH conditions, however, choose to access the BH sector for assessment and treatment.(P. S. Wang, Berglund, et al.,

2005) Most patients with BH problems are seen in the physical health sector where few BH practitioners are present to assist primary and specialty medical clinicians in the delivery of outcome changing BH care. This we refer to as the BH specialist-BH patient mismatch (Figure 11-2).

Figure 11-2. BH Specialist-BH Patient Mismatch

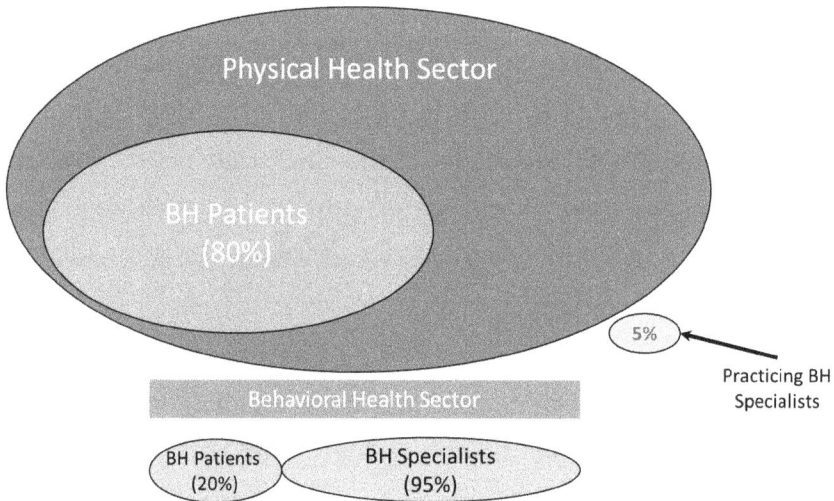

The original intent in creating a standalone BH sector was to maximize delivery of evidencebased care to patients in most need of BH interventions in settings designed for such. Unfortunately, few of those who need BH services have been or are willing to access treatment in independent BH service locations. This includes the majority of patients with serious and persistent behavioral conditions, albeit with the possible exception of patients with schizophrenia. Those who do choose to seek assistance for their BH conditions in the BH sector find that there are often delays of six or more weeks before initial appointments can be made due to personnel shortages.(Cunningham, 2009) Timely follow-up can pose a challenge for the same reason. Hindered access is particularly problematic for those with limited financial resources or those in public programs.

BH Sector Delivery of Care

The BH sector provides services in a different way than all other specialty medical settings. First, it is supported through funding streams segregated from all other medical disciplines (to be covered later). Separate payment procedures sometimes create the requirement to place service locations at a distance from other general medical and specialty services. This occurs either directly, as a part of participation rules, or indirectly by decrements in the amount paid for services or the complicated procedures needed to obtain permission to provide them. These BH service locations are governed by an independent set of regulatory and fiscal rules that create challenges in delivering coordinated care to patients, and especially to those with concurrent medical and BH conditions.

Second, clinicians that treat patients in the BH sector participate in networks of providers that may be independent from all other medical providers. Thus, they are responsive to needs delineated by the BH sector service locations (and payers), including where services can be delivered, to whom, and with what type of BH professionals. Further, they often maintain independent record keeping and quality improvement systems even when colleagues from other medical specialties working for the same hospital and clinic system also see the patients for whom they care. Communication among medical and BH practitioners can be difficult and in some situations impossible. In addition, independent record keeping prevents analysis of total health outcomes for patients with both medical and BH care needs.

Finally, despite the frequency with which patients with concurrent medical and BH conditions are seen, in many cases the BH sector is designed only for the delivery of BH care, often to the exclusion of any medical interventions other than the most basic. Conversely, the medical setting avoids delivery of BH services since they are considered the responsibility of professionals in the BH sector (and paid through a separate budget). This creates significant problems in medical and BH emergency rooms (ERs), in acute medical and BH settings (hospitals), in post-acute care settings (nursing home and assisted living facilities), and in medical and BH outpatient clinics.

Five to ten percent of "medical" ER visits are for patients with primary BH conditions.(Larkin, Claassen, Emond, Pelletier, & Camargo, 2005) Additionally, up to 40% of patients with a primary medical reason for their ER visits have a BH comorbidity contributing to the patient's health need, such as substance abuse associated with auto accidents and falls.(Richmond et al., 2007) Despite these statistics, medical ERs typically do not have psychiatrist coverage, virtually the only allopathic medical specialty overlooked for ER participation. Likewise, standalone BH emergency assessment facilities, primarily accessible in standalone psychiatric facilities, have no medical service capabilities. Such segregation of services is associated with up to 25% higher BH-related admission rates to both medical and BH units and a high use of ambulances to transport patients from BH to medical ERs, and vice versa, for cross-disciplinary assessments.

In acute general hospital (GH) settings, consistently 25% to 35% of general medical admissions have BH comorbidity (Table 11-1). One would expect that such a high frequency would necessitate support for inpatient BH services access; however, BH specialists and clinical settings with medical and BH capabilities are the exception rather than the rule. Medical and psychiatric units, even if located in the same GH, are configured for discipline-specific care. Psychiatric units cannot handle acute medical problems and medical units address BH comorbidity only if it becomes flagrant, requiring physical or chemical restraints, one-on-one supervision, or transfer for close observation in the intensive care unit. Even then, cross-disciplinary patient treatment is not part of the equation in either setting. Transfers or safety measures prior to transfer are most typically provided.

Table 11-1. General Hospital Medical Admissions* with BH Comorbidity

Core Delivery Systems	Number of Hospitals	Total Adm/Yr	% BH	Longer BH vs. non-BH ALOS	Higher BH vs. non-BH Readmits	Sitter Use
System 1	>10	135,000+	26%	1.1	30%	$6.0M
System 2	1	19,000+	36%	1.2	40%	$3.1M
System 3	4	34,500+	29%	1.3	70%	$.42M
System 4	5	40,000+	26%	1.8	30%	$2+M
System 5	1	16,000+	23%	0.6	45%	

*Medical and surgical admissions to five general hospital systems in the US, excluding neonate and primary psychiatric admissions.

Separation of medical and BH services even occurs in post-acute settings. BH providers build support services at selected nursing facilities that are independent of medical services, even for patients in whom both medical and BH issues contribute to challenges in assisting them with health needs. This limits the ability of post-acute settings to accept comorbid patients from acute care settings. Even though acute medical and BH conditions have stabilized enough for discharge, post-acute cross-disciplinary needs can lead to extended delays in placement to lower levels of care.

The last disconnect in medical and BH service is in outpatient clinics. Half of patients with serious mental illness have one or more chronic medical condition,(Druss & Walker, 2011) whereas BH comorbidity is present in 30% of medical outpatients.(Druss & Walker, 2011) As in the GH setting, access to coordinated outpatient medical and BH care is typically not available in either the primary medical or BH setting. The disconnect in medical and BH service coordination is now becoming a recognized area of potential growth due to the high clinical and economic cost of comorbidity. Neither the medical nor the BH settings have found ways to effectively introduce outcome changing, value-added, cross-disciplinary services because of funding challenges.

As a result, low cost BH professionals, such as counselors and social workers, are hired to assist with BH issues in medical settings because budget work arounds can often support their addition. However, they have limited assessment and intervention capabilities, especially for high cost patients with complex health conditions, including treatment resistant BH issues. Use of low cost BH professionals is not associated with either improved long-term clinical or fiscal outcomes.(Bower, Knowles, Coventry, & Rowland, 2011) On the reverse side, medical practitioners added to BH settings find that they are limited in their medical assessments since simple and available ancillary medical testing and procedures are not possible in BH settings devoted to delivery of targeted BH services.

This mismatch of patients, providers, and settings is associated with well-documented adverse health outcomes. Medical patients with largely untreated comorbid BH conditions (1) are medical ilness treatment resistant, (2) experience persistent medical symptoms and more chronic illness complications, (3) report greater impairment, (4) use more disability days, and (5) have doubling of total health care costs when compared to medical patients without BH comorbidity.(R. Kathol et al., 2005; W. J. Katon & Seelig, 2008; Prince et al., 2007; Seelig & Katon, 2008) Unfortunately, parity laws do not improve access to BH services in the medical setting nor does the Affordable Care Act. They merely state that BH services should be "available" and paid *on par* with similar medical services. Nothing assures where and how they should be delivered, such as in the medical setting.

The Effect of Siloed Payments for BH Services on Medical and BH Care Delivery

Most non-BH clinicians and medical adminstrators are unaware of the effect that segregated payment for BH services has on their patients' access to evidence-based BH and medical care. Even medical health plan executives do not understand that "carving-out" or "carving-in" BH benefits from their medical insurance products significantly limits the ability of medical and BH practitioners to deliver coordinated care.

Segregated BH Payment Practices

Prior to passage of the ACA, health plans and the purchasers of their products were the primary organizations at risk for the total cost of care in covered populations. Further, while capitated contracts were occasionally used, the majority of contracts for medical care were based on fee-for-service business practices (i.e., volume-based). Thus, health plans and self-insured employers attempted to create payment practices designed to support delivery of services while controlling costs. Using volume-based models, payment practices often fostered delivery of unnecessary services while preventing delivery of value-added services, especially to those with complex health conditions and exceedingly high health care service use.

The ACA has created a new dynamic in the marketplace. Networks of treating clinicians (e.g., doctors) have become fiscally accountable for the quality and cost-effective delivery of value-added services. They are expected to use their understanding of health and health care delivery to develop coordinated delivery approaches that improve the patient experience, lead to better health, and save money to help meet the Triple Aim objective of the Medicare Shared Savings Program (MSSP). As a part of the ACA MSSP initiative, networks of providers (e.g., ACOs) in alliance with various other stakeholders in the health care delivery system (e.g., health plans, employers, government agencies, hospitals and clinics), are building new delivery approaches and payment practices to foster efficient and effective care. If successful, and quality thresholds are met, treatment providers can share in associated savings. Importantly, some of these networks are also at-risk for negative health and cost outcomes. This new "pay-for-performance" model we refer to as the "ACO World."

Under the historic fee-for-service model of care delivery and payment, health plans and payers instituted various utilization management initiatives in an attempt to monitor and reduce risk, thereby controlling costs. Among these initiatives has been the establishment of managed care organizations (MCOs) and separate managed behavioral health organizations (MBHOs). In these situations, separate medical and BH funding pools independently pay for medical and BH professional services and facility costs, which persists even after passage of the ACA (Figure 11-3).

Figure 11-3. Siloed Payment for Medical and BH Services Even in the ACO World

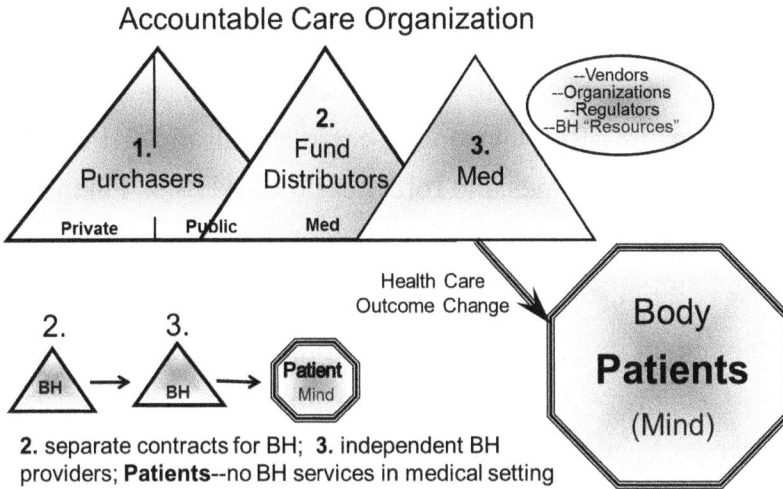

When a MCO "owns" its own BH business, funding for BH care uniformly comes from a BH subsidiary of the MCO plan. This BH subsidiary is known as a MBHO "carve-in." Alternatively, a medical health plan can choose to buy management of their BH business from an independent MBHO vendor. This is known as an MBHO "carve-out." Regardless of whether BH business is carved-in or carved-out, budgets for BH care are distinct from those for medical care. Importantly, the medical and BH budgets may compete with each other so that each can maximize profits from the populations they serve, even if the populations are the same.

While conceptually, one would think that carve-ins would be more supportive of BH services delivery, in fact, many carve-ins are more aggressive in managing (or minimizing) BH services utilization than some carve-outs. Both carve-ins and carve-outs have a vested interest in channeling payment for BH services from their budgets to their medical payment counterparts, especially when non-network "medical" providers in medical settings provide them. While the opportunity is present for carve-ins to look at the interaction of medical and BH costs for the same covered patients, this rarely happens since patient identifiers are separate, claims adjudication often occurs in discrete servers, and few understand the important impact that concurrent medical and BH conditions have on clinical outcomes and total health care costs. Furthermore, MBHOs benefit by isolating the BH payment system. They have no incentive to integrate benefits or services.

Independent budgets carry with them an additional feature. Since BH coverage is separate from all other medical services, purchasers of health care for selected populations, such as employers or government programs, can choose to purchase medical and BH care for their enrollees from different vendors. Thus, an employer could contract with Health Plan A to pay for medical services for its employees and with MBHO B (a carved-out MBHO) for BH services. This creates a disconnect for patients and providers since the practitioners providing medical care through the Health Plan A's contract benefits may work in the same system as BH providers, but the BH providers contract with Health Plan A's MBHO, Health Plan A's BH carve-in, and not with MBHO B.

Disconnects such as this are common and lead to the need for medical providers to suggest that patients call a "1-800" number to access a BH professional rather than sending the patient down the hall to a known BH in-network colleague, as commonly occurs with pulmonary, surgical, or pediatric colleagues in the same "network" of providers. The situation becomes even more complicated when independent medical and BH payers cover patients needing medical and BH care. When a patient has medical coverage for services in one health system, but BH coverage for network services in a competing health system, both patients and practitioners suffer from the necessary disconnect. Alternatively, the patient can absorb additional costs of non-network treatment. More often, however, the patient and medical practitioner merely choose to ignore the BH condition with the resultant outcomes noted above.

Practice of BH in an Independent Payment System

Independent payment for BH and medical services shows up at multiple levels within the health care system (Table 11-2). First, it creates a competitive environment between medical and BH care delivery since each system is responsible for supporting services while maximizing profits from the discipline-specific services for which they are responsible. It does not matter that the BH budget for direct BH care constitutes only two to seven percent of the total health care spend (discussed below). Each looks to the most efficient use of its own resources, concentrating exclusively on those for which it is accountable.

Table 11-2. Effect of Independent Medical and BH Payment on Health System, Insurer, and Clinical Care Factors

	Factors	Effects
Health System	Interaction of medical and BH systems	Little communication, including EHR
Insurers	Patient identifiers	Two identifiers
	Payment pool	Two buckets
	Contract benefit descriptions	Disparate coverage and rules
	Network of providers	Separate medical and BH
	Member and provider support	Separate call-in numbers
	Approval process	Separate rules & approaches

	Factors	Effects
	Case & utilization management	Discipline-specific
	Coding, billing, claims adjudication	Separate payment rules and billing forms
	Data warehousing & actuarial analysis	Separate & discrete
	Quality improvement programs	Discipline-specific
Clinical Care	Practice locations	Paid independently; necessarily separate
	Services delivery	Segregated
	Clinician collaboration and communication	Rare

Second, a separate budget for BH services necessitates duplication of health plan administrative divisions, such as those listed in Table 2. Carve-outs do this naturally since they are independent companies and are required to support their insurance products through appropriate business practices. Interestingly, however, the same completely segregated divisions and work processes are also necessary for carve-ins, though owned by a single company. Thus, separate medical and BH budgets are also associated with considerably higher total health plan administrative costs.

Just like carve-outs, many carve-ins sell their BH products independent of the medical products sold by the same insurer. Thus, they require separate actuarial projections, patient identifiers, and a detached network of providers. Discrete benefit descriptions, member and provider support services, insurance approval processes, denial and appeals procedures, case and utilization management practices, and quality improvement programs follow from these. Since medical and BH budgets are isolated, then coding, billing, and claims adjudication disconnected from medical are also necessary. Logically, accumulated data from services supported by each would flow into segregated data warehouses, contributing to independently analyzed discipline-specific performance assessment and quality improvement programs.

Third, and perhaps most important, independent payment drives where and how BH services are delivered. The independent network of BH providers allows MBHOs to target payment only to those with credentials to provide BH services. Since facility fees are also generated as a part of the care delivery process, MBHOs typically require that BH services be provided in locations discrete from medical services. This not only focuses BH funds for BH care, but also prevents the potential for inadvertent payment for direct or ancillary medical services delivered to the same patients, who often have concurrent medical conditions.

Thus, while a separate payment system for BH conditions seems innocuous, in fact, it has pervasive effects on the ability of BH clinicians to practice in the medical setting. MBHOs are rigorous about making sure that their dollars go to BH care. The best and most financially successful means to do this is to ensure segregation of medical from BH services. It is these business practices that are associated with the "traditional" approach to BH care delivery described below. One can only imagine what our health care would look like if similar practices were used in the medical setting (i.e., managed pulmonary organizations (MPOs) or managed surgical organizations (MSOs) that independently handled service support and payment for patients with lung or surgical disease).

Clinical and Economic Consequences of Siloed Medical and Behavioral Health Payment Practices

Few stakeholders participating in the development of CINs and ACOs give much thought to the inclusion of BH practitioners and services as they build their integrated programs. Both MH and SUD services have traditionally been considered outside the purview of the rest of medical care. This perception, and the stigma that accompanies it, is perpetuated by the way that it is handled in the current medical environment.

Patients with BH conditions are treated in separate clinical locations. BH providers are members of separate networks of clinicians. Separate payers adjudicate payment for BH services. Treatment outcomes and costs are analyzed separately from medical outcomes and costs. Some even continue to think that BH conditions are not "real" illnesses; that those with BH disorders bring it on themselves, such as with SUDs; and that BH treatments are ineffective and unnecessarily costly.

Even for those who recognize the importance of BH comorbidity in medical patients on health and cost outcomes and the advances in BH treatment that lead to comparable outcomes as found in the medical setting, critical factors inhibit implementation of integrated BH and medical care as a part of CINs and ACOs. The most important factor is the siloed payment system described above. Unless this is changed, the integration of medical and BH services will, at best, be piecemeal with corresponding adverse consequences for the patient. The question is whether there is good reason for developing CINs, and especially those anticipating entering the full risk market, such as ACOs, to go to the effort to include BH providers and services as a core component of their clinical operations.

The best place to start addressing this question is by taking a look at the financial impact that patients with BH conditions have on health care spending. In a recent report produced for the American Psychiatric Association, Melek et al(Melek, Norris, & Paulus, 2013) at Milliman, Inc. used available commercial, Medicare, and Medicaid health care databases to assess health care costs for individuals with and without BH comorbidity covered by these three insurance vehicles. Consistent with other literature, their report confirmed that at a national level, the total cost of care for patients with BH conditions was 2.5 to 3.5 times that of those with no BH condition. Medicaid BH patients had 3.4 times the cost of those without (per member per month [PMPM] $1,301 versus $381). BH patients covered by commercial insurance or Medicare were 2.8 and 2.4 times more expensive, respectively (PMPM $940 versus $340 and $1,404 versus $582, respectively).

Also consistent with the literature, the majority of what's spent for BH patients was for medical services, with a range of 71% (Medicaid) to 92% (Medicare). In fact, if one compares the total spend for BH services in those with BH conditions to the "medical" spend (Table 11-3), the medical spend is nearly five times higher than the BH spend. This finding is magnified if one considers that nearly half of the BH spend for commercial and Medicaid patients was for BH medications (data not available for Medicare patients). Primary care physicians, not psychiatrists, write most BH prescriptions.

Table 11-3. Is BH the "Bottomless Pit"?

	Total Population Served	% of Pop. with BH Claims	Total Annual Spend	BH* Spend	Total Medical Claims Incurred by BH Pop. (% of Medical Claims
Commercial	198.8M	14%	$1.0T	$42.9B	$275B (28.7%)

	Total Population Served	% of Pop. with BH Claims	Total Annual Spend	BH* Spend	Total Medical Claims Incurred by BH Pop. (% of Medical Claims
Medicare/ Medicaid	91.8M	9%/20%	$0.67T	$49.0B	$169B (26.3%)
Total	290.6M	14%	$1.7T	$91.9B	$444B (27.5%)

*Includes BH meds for commercial and Medicaid but not Medicare.

Health plan claims data confirms that the addition of BH comorbidity in patients with medical conditions increases the total annual cost of care. This is readily evident in a consolidation of claims data on a nationally representative population of nearly six million patients covered by public and private insurance products performed by Cartesian Solutions, Inc.™ (Table 11-4). In this Table, the presence of a chronic medical illness doubles the annual cost of care compared to the entire population. In the thirty to forty percent with concurrent BH conditions and a chronic medical illness, annual cost of care more than doubles again.

Table 11-4. Health and Cost Impact of BH Comorbidity in Patients with Chronic Medical Conditions

Patient Groups	Annual Cost of Care	Illness Prevalence	% with Comorbid BH Condition*	Annual Cost with BH Condition	% Increase with BH Condition
All insured	$2,920		15%		
Arthritis	$5,220	6.6%	36%	$10,710	94%
Asthma	$3,730	5.9%	35%	$10,030	169%
Cancer	$11,650	4.3%	37%	$18,870	62%
Diabetes	$5,480	8.9%	30%	$12,280	124%
CHF	$9,770	1.3%	40%	$17,200	76%
Migraine	$4,340	8.2%	43%	$10,810	149%
COPD	$3,840	8.2%	38%	$10,980	186%

Cartesian Solutions, Inc.™--consolidated health plan claims data
*Approximately 10% receive evidence-based mental condition treatment.

These national findings are also reflected in what is experienced at the care delivery system level. Table 11-1 indicates that the 25% to 35% of patients admitted to medical and surgical units in general hospitals with comorbid BH conditions, excluding those admitted for primary psychiatric conditions, had longer average lengths of stay and higher readmission rates, both indicators of high total health care costs. The predominance of high medical versus BH costs in medical patients with comorbid BH conditions is further clarified in a Truven MarketScan database analysis where employees and their covered dependents with diabetes mellitus and alcoholism had PMPM costs of care 2.2 times higher than those without (Table 11-5). Ninety-one percent of the costs for those with comorbid alcoholism were for medical services and non-BH medications.   These findings are similar to another population of patients with diabetes and depression.

Table 11-5. Diabetes – The Impact of Alcoholism

Chronic Medical Condition: DIABETES	Annual Episode Rate per 1,000	Average Number of Services Per Episode	Annual Utilization Rate per 1,000	Average Allowed Cost per Unit	Average Paid Cost per Unit	Paid Cost Per Member Per Month
with Alcoholism						
IP Facility-BHV	187.34	4.63	868.12	$757.63	$665.92	$48.17
IP Facility-MED	607.39	6.62	4,021.93	$1,475.13	$1,453.99	$487.32
PHP/IOP	187.82	7.48	1,405.02	$233.21	$206.46	$24.17
Hosp ER/Lab/Rad/Oth	2,481.24	17.65	43,784.51	$195.99	$168.01	$613.00
OP Professional-BHV	320.60	11.23	3,599.94	$82.11	$61.66	$18.50
Prof/Other Medical	8,082.01	8.11	65,570.54	$90.54	$78.80	$430.56
RX Behavioral			11,843.22	$88.74	$73.99	$73.02
RX Medical			30,931.70	$88.96	$72.99	$188.13
TOTAL	**166.84**	**13.65**	**2,278.06**	**$157.60**	**$139.45**	**$1,882.88**
w/o Alcoholism						
IP Facility-BHV	3.99	6.79	27.09	$659.62	$548.08	$1.24
IP Facility-MED	178.46	6.07	1,083.34	$1,392.35	$1,335.05	$120.53
PHP/IOP	7.56	4.57	34.55	$185.84	$157.01	$0.45
Hosp	1,536.06	12.22	18,773.11	$199.65	$169.82	$265.67

Chronic Medical Condition: DIABETES	Annual Episode Rate per 1,000	Average Number of Services Per Episode	Annual Utilization Rate per 1,000	Average Allowed Cost per Unit	Average Paid Cost per Unit	Paid Cost Per Member Per Month
ER/Lab/Rad/Oth						
OP Professional BHV	61.57	8.36	514.55	$83.72	$59.49	$2.55
Prof/Other Medical	7,315.85	5.88	43,007.41	$83.95	$68.88	$246.88
RX Behavioral	-	-	4,443.18	$84.12	$68.79	$25.47
RX Medical	-	-	31,317.00	$92.58	$74.33	$193.99
TOTAL	11,302.64	10.90	123,164.27	$123.06	$103.64	$856.77

The data analyses performed by Melek et al and Cartesian Solutions, Inc.™ provide robust support for the fact that BH comorbidity is associated with high health care service use. The majority of this is for medical not BH service. In fact, earlier sections in this Chapter on the delivery of BH care indicate that BH care has limited availability in the medical setting and that patients with BH conditions seen in the medical setting don't accept referral to the BH sector. This is consistent with findings in the literature that most with BH conditions seen in the medical setting go untreated.(P. S. Wang et al., 2007; P. S. Wang, Lane, et al., 2005)

The lack of treatment for BH conditions in the medical setting is associated not only with poor BH outcomes, but it also predicts that patients, such as those with diabetes and depression, will have more symptoms. Patients will respond worse to treatment, will have worse medical illness control and more complications, will have less satisfaction with medical care, will be more disabled, and will have higher mortality than patients with medical illness alone.(Chang et al., 2011; Druss, Zhao, Von Esenwein, Morrato, & Marcus, 2011) Untreated BH conditions in medical patients have more than just cost consequences. They are also associated with greater impairment and persistent, poorly treated medical illness.

Thus, we come back to the comments at the beginning of this section. Does it make sense that BH services and providers should become core members of CINs as they are conceptualized and built? Since CINs or ACOs are tasked with putting together services that will lead to health improvement and conservation of health resources, then inclusion of BH providers and services as essential features seems reasonable. This, however, is only true if the addition of BH providers in the medical setting add value by improving health and cost outcomes.

Further, current payment practices and resultant care delivery processes do nothing to encourage greater consideration for the inclusion of BH services and professionals as core participants in CINs and ACOs. For instance, BH providers are paid exclusively by MBHOs. This necessarily creates a challenge for organizations setting up CINs and ACOs since they would then be required to set up payment work arounds that allow BH providers to deliver services to medical patients with BH comorbidity. The next sections discuss strategies to support value-added, non-traditional BH services through CINs and ACOs while transitioning from segregated to integrated medical and BH benefit contracting.

Models of Value-Added BH Care

The United States currently lives in a world of what we will call "traditional" BH service delivery. As discussed in the Section on BH Sector Delivery of Care, above, traditional BH services are almost exclusively provided in the BH sector. While this can help BH patients willing to avail themselves of treatment there, it is of no use to the seventy to eighty percent of BH patients seen exclusively or primarily in the medical sector. Restricting treatment to the BH setting also limits communication between BH providers and medical providers, an important aspect of coordinated care since medical and BH illnesses interact.

If BH professionals practicing in the BH sector are characteristic of traditional BH, then "non-traditional" BH may be characterized by delivery of BH services in the medical setting. The first attempt to do this was to add BH care to primary and specialty medical physicians' list of tasks for which they were responsible. It is no wonder that this path of least cost has not succeeded. Primary care physicians are already burdened with a 150% time commitment in a 100% time world just to provide for preventive, acute and chronic medical care needs.(Ostbye et al., 2005; Yarnall, Pollak, Ostbye, Krause, & Michener, 2003) Specialty medical physicians, also busy, are encumbered by limited interest in becoming involved in emotions, cognitions, and behavior when their preferred attention targets their chosen specialty area. To time and interest constraints, there is also the fact that primary and specialty medical physicians have limited training in evidence-based application of BH interventions, especially in medical patients with chronic and complex illness.

In order for the introduction of BH services in the primary and specialty medical setting to succeed, it is necessary for BH specialists with skills, time, and interest in the area to join medical teams and contribute to the holistic care of patients. It is unlikely, however, that the ninety-plus percent of BH practitioners working in the BH sector are going to put on their marching shoes and move to the medical sector to practice. They still get paid for providing services in the traditional BH setting, and this is unlikely to change soon.

An alternative would be for primary care and specialty medical system profits to pay for BH specialists to treat patients in the medical setting. This scenario is an equally unlikely possibility since primary care practices also have financial challenges. Specialty medical services are reluctant for both economic and perceptual reasons. They, after all, are primarily accountable only for specialty service outcomes.

Even if there were a way to pay for low cost counselors or social workers, would this be a value-added addition in the primary and specialty medical setting? A recent Cochrane review of counselor use in the UK, i.e., professionals who provide similar services to counselors and social workers in the United States, suggests not. While there was short-term satisfaction, there were no improved long-term clinical outcomes or cost savings,(Bower et al., 2011; Bower, Rowland, & Hardy, 2003) even after 40 years of implementation adjustments and outcome assessments.

Value-Added BH

For purposes of this Chapter, we use the term "value-added" to denote clinical services that have the potential to improve health and lower cost when delivered to a population of patients. This concept is core to the development of CINs and ACOs and should be no different for BH services than other decisions being made when setting up a CIN and/or ACO.

If traditional BH services are not an option for adding value for patients, since they do not target patients in the medical setting nor coordinate medical and BH service delivery, what about non-traditional BH services? During the past twenty years, there are a number of non-traditional approaches to BH care that show substantial promise (Table 11-6). Some have irrefutable data showing that when they are introduced, predictable improvements in health and cost occur.

Table 11-6. Examples of Value-Added Non-Traditional BH and Medical Services

(Improves Outcomes and Lowers Cost)

Category	Description
Depression and diabetes	2 months fewer days of depression/year; project $2.9 million/year lower total health costs/100,000 diabetic members[1]
Panic disorder in PC	2 months fewer days of anxiety/year; project $1.7 million/year lower total health costs/100,000 diabetic members[2]
Substance use disorders with medical compromise	14% increase in abstinence; $2,050 lower annual health care cost/patient in integrated program[3]
Delirium prevention programs	30% lower incidence of delirium; projected $16.5 million/year reduction in IP costs/30,000 admissions[4]
Unexplained physical complaints	no increase in missed general medical illness or adverse events; 9% to 53% decrease in costs associated with increased healthcare service utilization[5]
Health complexity	halved depression prevalence; statistical improvement of quality of life, perceived physical and mental health; 7% reduction in new admissions at 12 months[6]
Proactive psychiatric consultation	doubled psychiatric involvement with .92 shorter ALOS and 4:1 to 14:1 return on investment[7]

Notes: 1. Katon et al, *Diab Care* 29:265-270, 2006; 2. Katon et al, *Psychological Med* 36:353-363, 2006; 3. Parthasarathy et al, *Med Care* 41:257-367, 2003; 4. Inouye et al, Arch Int Med 163:958-964, 2003; 5. summary of 8 experimental/control outcome studies; 6. Stiefel et al, *Psychoth Psychosom* 77:247, 2008; 7. Desan et al, P*sychosom* 52:513, 2011.

Perhaps the best studied is the collaborative care model for depression identification and treatment in medical patients.(W. Katon et al., 2012; W. J. Katon et al., 2010; Unutzer et al., 2012; Unutzer et al., 2008; Woltmann et al., 2012) Over seventy randomized trials now confirm that a stepped approach to the care of depression in the primary care setting will improve depression and lower total cost of care in those exposed. Cost savings accrue for up to five years after exposure to the intervention and can be associated with millions of dollars in savings for populations as small as 100,000. More recent studies, in which the care managers who previously focused on support for depression treatment expanded their assistance to include concurrent medical conditions, now show that clinical improvement of associated chronic medical conditions can also occur with augmented depression outcomes in what is now called TEAMCare.(W. J. Katon et al., 2010)

While less well studied, there are also a number of non-traditional models of BH delivery that have initial data and significant promise since inpatient care is so much more expensive than outpatient care (Table 11-7). The two models with the best data are delirum prevention programs and proactive psychiatric consultation services. In the former, a BH team works with medical hospitalist clinicians to identify and correct anticedents to the development of delirium in at-risk patients. Several studies show that delirium prevention programs can decrease the occurance of delirium by one-third. Since delirium is associated with doubling of hospitalization days, both decreased morbidity and cost savings can be expected.

Table 11-7. Examples of Value-Added Non-Traditional Programs

Examples
• Inpatient and outpatient--complexity-based integrated care/case management
• Inpatient
○ General hospital emergency room psychiatrist coverage and treatment capability
○ Proactive psychiatry consultation teams
○ Delirium prevention and treatment programs
○ Standardized protocols for common BH situations in medical settings
○ Constant observation (sitter/security guard) review
○ Complexity Intervention Units (CIUs) with PH and BH capabilities in general hospitals
• Outpatient
○ Onsite TEAMCare services--includes all medical and BH conditions for complex patients
○ Functional symptom training and support
○ Substance use disorder assessment and treatment programs,

Examples
including buprenorphine and SBIRT
• Post-acute care--nursing homes with medical and BH coverage & capabilities

The proactive psychiatric consultation model assigns members of a BH team, led by a psychiatrist, to work with admitting hospitalists from the day of a patient's medical admission. These proactive consultants identify BH comorbidities that prevent improvement in patients' medical conditions or are associated with extended hospital stays.(Desan, Zimbrean, Weinstein, Bozzo, & Sledge, 2011) Using this model, it has been shown that average length of stay (ALOS) for affected patients can be reduced by one to three days depending on how patients are targeted and assistance is given. Again, this is a model with promise.

Other less well studied models of non-traditional BH care, include the introduction of psychiatrists in medical emergency rooms,(Little-Upah et al., 2013; Lucas et al., 2009) the development of Complexity Intervention Units,(R. G. Kathol et al., 2009) delirium treatment programs,(Akunne, Murthy, & Young, 2012; Chen et al., 2011; Inouye, Bogardus, Williams, Leo-Summers, & Agostini, 2003; W. Wang et al., 2012) development of common BH problem protocols (e.g., substance withdrawal, agitation/delirium) for use in medical settings, review of sitter (one-on-one patient supervision) use, and adding integrated case managers to support treatment for complex patients.(R. Kathol, Perez, & Cohen, 2010) Each of these has sufficient preliminary data to support their serious consideration as value-added programs are introduced into medical settings.

When to Introduce Value-Added BH Programs in CINs and ACOs

The first question to consider when deciding whether BH professionals should participate as core members of a CIN or ACO relates to the population served and the impact that BH conditions might have on health and cost outcomes. Virtually all advanced CINs, also called ACOs, would benefit from BH professional participation as full network member providers. ACOs may be at full-risk for total health outcomes and costs of the populations that they serve. Only by including BH professionals in their network will they have the opportunity to capture savings by decreasing unnecessary medical service use as BH conditions come under control.

By having BH providers as part of the CIN/ACO network, the BH providers will have the same expectations as all other network providers. They will attend the same indoctrination sessions; utilize the same clinical documentation, communication, and outcome recording approaches; implement the same quality care guidelines; follow the same referral and network program use parameters; have performance judged by the same outcome metrics as other providers in the ACO, and have their outcomes analyzed within consolidated medical and BH findings. Most importantly, however, network BH providers will adopt the primary goals of the ACO (i.e., to maximize total health outcomes and efficient use of resources for patients treated among the populations served). They would also be incented to apply effective and efficient medical practices, similar to other network providers, in order to share in ACO profits (or losses).

Since thirty to forty percent of medical patients served by an ACO have high health costs associated with comorbid BH conditions, in-network BH professionals, deployed in value-added

BH programs in the medical setting, can work as health care team members with medical providers to improve health and thereby attenuate cost. If BH providers are not ACO members, on the other hand, either the ACO would have to create economic incentives for the BH providers to work in the medical setting or the BH providers would be forced to continue to provide traditional BH services paid on a siloed, fee-for-service basis, which bring no value to the ACO where the BH need is greatest.

The need for BH specialists to participate in more basic CINs (i.e., those delivering focused health services for a target population, such as a CIN of cardiologists or gastroenterologists, a CIN for pain management, a CIN specializing in rehabilitation, or a large primary care group practice CIN), would depend on the degree to which BH issues would contribute to health and cost outcomes for the target population. For instance, a targeted pain management CIN would serve a population with a high number of patients in whom untreated substance use disorders and depression predictably affects health and cost outcomes. BH specialists would logically contribute to improving health and lowering cost. BH issues would be less central to treatment in a cardiology CIN though a case for BH CIN provider participation could still be made since depression is now a known predictor of cardiac morbidity and mortality post-myocardial infarction.

After a decision is made about the need to include in-network BH professionals as core CIN providers, then the question arises about how to initiate the process (i.e., build or buy). The only BH purchase option in the market today is for traditional standalone BH services. Current BH providers only know this method of care delivery because it is the only one that allows fiscal (albeit marginal) solvency. To buy BH professionals and their services from existing vendors, even the ones that say they do "integrated care," therefore, will necessarily involve expansion of standalone BH care, a model consistent with the poor health and cost outcomes described above. Thus, the better option is to build the type of BH services that will bring the CIN/ACO value as it transitions to population-based risk contracting characteristic of health reform.

Building value-added BH services makes clinical and economic sense. By doing so, the CIN can hire and deploy BH professional teams configured to maximize clinical outcomes for medical patients with concurrent BH conditions, which lead to cost savings. Since the majority of patients are not currently receiving BH services in the medical setting, they will experience a better treatment encounter (patient centered approach). They will have improved health outcomes, presuming that evidence-based approaches to BH professional introduction are used. And, deployed correctly, they should decrease the additional medical spend, which is where the majority of waste is present in their care.

So how does one initially build a value-added BH program in a CIN/ACO?

Strategy to Introduce Value-Added BH Programs in CINs and ACOs

As documented above, the prevalence of BH conditions in the medical setting is significant. Few, if any, care delivery systems have the resources necessary to support the introduction of the number of BH professionals needed to address all patients' needs, especially when 30% or more of any population is affected. Further, there are few BH providers practicing in the medical setting and even fewer that would know how to deliver value-added services. Thus, if a system did have the resources to retain the necessary BH expertise, recruitment and retention of the necessary personnel would be challenging. Nor would medical health plans be likely to expand reimbursement to cover all BH care in the medical setting, especially since management and payment of BH services is typically siloed elsewhere.

Thus, it becomes important that non-traditional integrated BH services be implemented in a way that maximizes benefit to the most needy and costly patients while establishing value-added programs that produce the best outcomes. Results from early efforts can guide program expansion. For this reason, strategic introduction of non-traditional BH "teams" to deliver value-added services described above *for targeted high risk, high cost medical patients* is best. By doing this, it is possible to support and surpass unmet salary requirements for the additional BH professionals from savings achieved by the reduction of total medical service use, thus providing justification through a return on investment.

At-risk patients can be identified through predictive modeling tools, claims databases, registries, or developed clinical algorithms. This should start with chronic and complex patients seen in various medical settings. (Parenthetically, there are also high risk, high cost primary BH patients in traditional BH settings who could be similarly targeted with successful health improvement and reduction in total cost of care, but the scope of this Chapter does not allow elaboration on this topic.) Once identified, such patients could then be served by the value-added, non-traditional BH services described above.

Implementation of Integrated BH Services

Figure 11-4 summarizes the current state of ACO development as it relates to use of BH services; the impacts of current-state care delivery procedures on patients, outcomes, and costs; and the recommended transition process to a value-added future state. While each CIN/ACO will design a future state gauged to its mission, vision, and goals; ultimately, the desired outcome is the creation of a CIN/ACO that maximizes health while conserving delivery system resources in a patient-friendly system. It is necessary, however, to stage the transition in a way that financially supports health systems going from fee-for-service contracting to risk-based global contracting for services. We will discuss one approach that can be taken.

Figure 11-4. BH ACO Service Delivery
(Current to Future State)

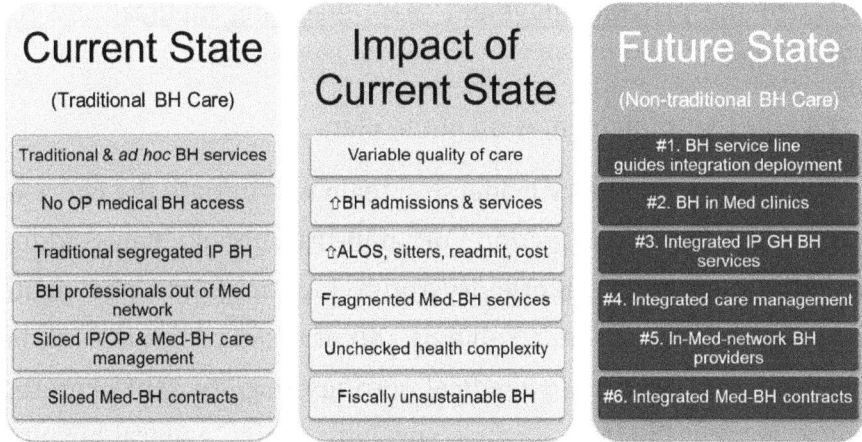

Current State (Traditional BH Care)	Impact of Current State	Future State (Non-traditional BH Care)
Traditional & *ad hoc* BH services	Variable quality of care	#1. BH service line guides integration deployment
No OP medical BH access	⇧BH admissions & services	#2. BH in Med clinics
Traditional segregated IP BH	⇧ALOS, sitters, readmit, cost	#3. Integrated IP GH BH services
BH professionals out of Med network	Fragmented Med-BH services	#4. Integrated care management
Siloed IP/OP & Med-BH care management	Unchecked health complexity	#5. In-Med-network BH providers
Siloed Med-BH contracts	Fiscally unsustainable BH	#6. Integrated Med-BH contracts

The first step (#1) for many organizations will entail the development of a non-traditional BH Service Line. For instance, one medical and one BH thought leader within an organization could co-chair a cross-disciplinary, multi-professional task force charged with designing and deploying standardized BH service in the medical setting. Specifically, CIN leadership of the BH Service Line will want to:

- Design a clear vision for medical/BH integration,

- Identify/quantify existing barriers to achieving that vision,

- Determine the consequences of <u>not</u> making the necessary changes, i.e., doing nothing,

- Design the optimal service complement and degree of integration,

- Prioritize the services, providers, and populations to be addressed by the integration efforts,

- Design the implementation plan, including analytics for tracking successes and areas in need of strengthening,

- Design the provider payment plan, including medical and BH clinicians,

- Oversee the implementation of the plan.

This cross-disciplinary leadership team will initiate the chore of formulating the introduction of non-traditional, value-added integrated outpatient, emergency room, inpatient, and post-acute care programs (#2 and #3; Table 8). All of these programs will be embedded (co-located) in medical settings (e.g., patient-centered medical homes (PCMHs), medical specialty clinics, general hospital ERs, and inpatient medical units). They will have a functional relationship to traditional BH services but will be distinct in their operation.

In order to maximize the value brought to patients, providers, and the health system, integrated care/case managers (#4) will identify and assist, in collaboration with treating clinicians, the patients with the greatest complexity.(R. Kathol et al., 2010) This is the population present in all clinical settings that take the most clinical and administrative time, are the most challenging to treat, and use the most health care resources. Since 60% to 80% of these patients have comorbid BH problems,(Barnett et al., 2012) which if untreated predictably leads to poor outcomes, BH assessment and intervention, as a part of the care management process, is as important as medical.

BH professions providing services in the medical setting do not and will not meet salary demands in the current payment environment. In order to incentivize BH professionals to move to the medical setting and contribute to altering outcomes in complex comorbid patients, the best strategy is to include BH clinicians as part of the CIN/ACO network of providers (#5). By doing so, it will allow them to maximize the outcome changing BH expertise they bring as they integrate service delivery with other medical care. Perhaps more importantly, they can be supported in the service they provide under the guidance of the CIN/ACO rather than falling back on BH payment driven priorities. This will allow them to cover salary shortfalls via the savings generated through value-added care (covered below).

Finally, it is unsatisfactory and inappropriate for BH professionals contributing to better health outcomes and lower total costs of the population they serve to continue to have shortfalls in payment for services. To rectify this inequity, the final strategy for developing CINs/ACOs is to systematically move to contracting with medical health plans so that BH services delivered to the CIN/ACO network patients (#6; Figure 11-5) become a part of medical benefits. In essence, standalone contracts for BH payment by MBHOs, whether carve-ins or carve-outs, will sunset and will be picked up by the medical health plan. Such a transition is possible within three years of notification of intent to change contracting terms.

Figure 11-5. Recommended BH Strategy for BH Inclusion During ACO Formation

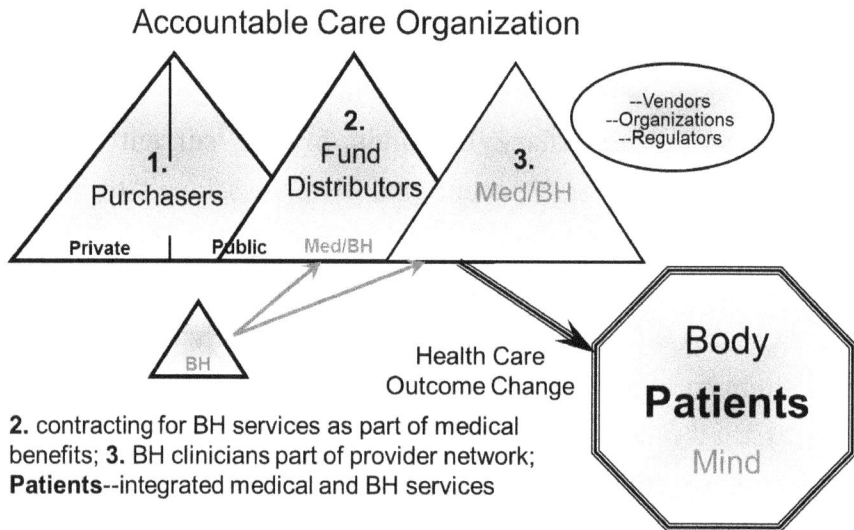

2. contracting for BH services as part of medical benefits; **3.** BH clinicians part of provider network; **Patients**--integrated medical and BH services

Traditional BH Services

The strategic inclusion of BH services by emerging CINs/ACOs described above focuses on building non-traditional BH service capabilities, but says little about how traditional BH providers and services will coordinate with them. Traditional BH service locations currently provide the majority of outcome changing services available to patients with BH disorders. Thus, this group of professionals will serve as an initial resource to newly developing non-traditional BH delivery capabilities. It is likely, however, that many of those presently working in tradtional settings will be re-deployed to medical settings where application of their expertise can bring greater value to needy and high cost BH patients and to the health system.

Only approximately 20% of BH patients are seen in the specialty BH setting. Many, but not most, of these have serious and persistent mental illnesses (SMIs) that require specialty BH services to meet their clinical needs. Traditional BH services in a specialty BH sector will, therefore, remain the primary service location for these patients. The specialty BH sector will also be a resource to BH patients increasingly treated in the medical sector for specialized BH treatments not likely to be available in many non-traditional BH locations (e.g., dialectical behavioral therapy (DBT), intensive outpatient programs (IOPs), electroconvulsive therapy (ECT), transcranial magnetic stimulation for depression, etc).

Many patients currently seen in the BH sector do not have a SMI or their SMI has stabilized to the point that they could be effectively treated in an expanded primary care-BH integrated service delivery setting. Thus, it is anticipated that over half of today's BH patients seen in the BH sector will transfer to the medical sector for treatment. This will become the default location in which evidence-based BH interventions are provided. This will allow them to be coordinated with evidence-based medical care. As this transition takes place, best practices coming from each discipline should be incorporated, such as the "recovery" approach used in the BH sector(Pratt, MacGregor, Reid, & Given, 2012) and cross-discplinary integrated case management technology, which assists with medical, BH, and non-clinical barriers to improvement without patient handoffs.(R. Kathol, Lattimer, Gold, Perez, & Gutteridge, 2011) Core components of the expanded non-traditional BH services are covered in a recent publication.(R.G. Kathol, deGruy, & Rollman, in press)

Ultimately, traditional BH services will be incorporated into non-tradtional BH work processes, both clinically and financially. A smaller and focused specialty BH sector will service the needs of difficult to control SMI and non-SMI patients. It will provide specialty expertise and capabilities only possible in a specialty BH service sector. The specialty BH sector, however, will have become a part of the medical delivery system.(Manderscheid & Kathol, in press) Benefits will be paid by medical insurance companies. BH providers will be part of medical networks, including CINs and ACOs. They will use common documentation systems and have the same expectations for proving delivery of outcome changing care. Further, medical services will be as available in specialty BH settings as in medical settings and paid from the same funding pool.

Most importantly, when SMI and challenging non-SMI patients stabilize, they will transfer back to the integrated non-traditional setting for continued care. In essence, non-traditional BH will decompress the backlog of patients having difficulty in accessing specialized services because less severe BH patients will be treated and followed in the primary care medical sector. It will be a collaborative relationship.

Opportunity Costs Related to BH Services in CINs/ACOs or the Costs of Doing Nothing

The authors of this Chapter have been working with employers, government agencies, health plans, and care delivery systems for the past twenty years. They have helped them explore the impact that BH conditions have on total health outcomes and cost. Until the ACA, however, there has been little interest in addressing the thorny issue of how to better handle BH care. Care delivery systems saw no need to become more efficient and effective in BH care delivery as long as they maintained financial stability or growth.

Interestingly, it is not the ACA but rather projections of national insolvency due to unbridaled medical costs that drive the need for change. The ACA is just the current vehicle being used to try to accomplish cost control while maintaining quality health. During the next decade, the U.S. health system will be expected to reign in medical inflation, which has consistently been two percentage points higher than the gross domestic product. Part of the solution will include changing the way that BH services are delivered and paid.

To date, there has been a disincentive for the health system to change the way that BH is supported and delivered. First, most consider that it represents only 2% to 7% of the total health care budget. This is hardly enough to require a revamp. Second, there are few health care professionals with either medical or BH administrative and clinical expertise that have a vision of what a revamped system would look like. Yet, it is clear that expanded traditional BH will bring little value.

Third, evidence indicates that untreated or ineffectively treated BH conditions, particularly in those with chronic medical conditions, leads to increased health service use (i.e., more admissions, longer lengths of stay, more ancillary testing, greater medication use, and increased numbers of specialty medical consultations). These are all areas of medicine that lead to financial success for stakeholders in delivering traditional, fee-for-service reimbursed care.

Health plans can demand higher premiums due to high service use. Hospitals and clinics can fill beds and clinic appointments. Pharmaceutical companies can sell more drugs. Device manufactures can sell more appliances. The only losers in the process are the purchasers of health care services and the patients. Interestingly, government purchasers are bigger losers than commercial insurers and large businesses since those with BH comorbidity are more likely to lose commercial coverage due to persistent health reasons and end up in public programs.

Population health, as a central component of the ACA, is now turning what used to be profitable areas of care delivery in the fee-for-service world, such as radiology departments, cardiac cath labs, orthopedic surgical suites, and long in-hospital stays, into cost centers. In order for CINs/ACOs taking risk to successfully compete for market share as a part of future risk-based contracting, care delivery systems must demonstrate the ability to reduce unnecessary service use, especially in specialty areas with high margins, and to document high quality care.

Thus, the emphasis is shifting to prevention and maximizing long-term outcomes for patients with high cost and unnecessary service use. It will no longer be advantageous for care delivery systems forming CINs and ACOs to ignore the negative impact that untreated or ineffectively treated BH comorbidity has on health and cost. They must learn ways to mitigate these negative effects so that fewer of their patients end up in what used to be their most profitable areas of service delivery.

The best way to start looking at the value that revamping BH service delivery would have on total health costs for populations served in a CIN/ACO is by reviewing the opportunity costs associated with the current tradtitional BH system (i.e., doing nothing). At a national level, more than $290 billion annually for additional medical costs in patients with BH disorders can be expected (Table 11-3). This is an unwieldy number, but doesn't tell us much about what happens at the care delivery level that leads to this number.

Table 11-5 gives a glimpse of where the extra spend for untreated or poorly treated BH patients in the medical setting occurs (i.e., in the medical inpatient and outpatient settings, in pharmaceutical use, and in ancillary medical service use). The amount spent for "BH services" in BH patients is one fifth the medical spend. Therefore, to the extent that expanded non-traditional BH services can efficiently and effectively reverse medical service use, CINs/ACOs can better compete as health reform progresses.

This is where "value-added" services come into play. Extra admissions, longer lengths of stay, professional fees, and ancillary services and medication use can be translated into dollars and cents (Table 11-8), as can the salary expense for strategically deployed non-traditional BH professionals. The trick is to customize BH professional deployment to the population served by each health system and geographic location so that delivery capabilities lead to population health and total health care cost reduction.

Table 11-8. ACO BH Transition Options

Options	Health Outcome	Cost Outcome
Do Nothing	• Poor BH access • Retarded medical illness improvement due to untreated BH comorbidity	• Unfavorable BH finances • Comorbid medical patients: ~1 day longer ALOS, >$M+ for sitters, ~30% higher 30-day readmissions; ~$M+ in extra service delivery costs
Traditional Standalone BH Expansion (Buy)	• ↑ BH access • Small impact on medical sector outcomes	• More unfavorable BH finances • Similar cost outcomes to above since value-added BH not possible in medical setting
BH Service Expansion into General Medical Service Area	• BH access in medical setting • Medical/BH provider communication; patient satisfaction • ↑ inpatient and outpatient care coordination and medical and BH outcomes	• Better payment for BH services from medical benefits • Gap closure on ALOS, sitter use, 30-day readmissions, cost/net margin for general medical patients with BH comorbidity

Table 11-6 shares calculations of documented cost savings or return on investment from published articles on value-added BH services introduced into the medical setting. If one uses these and other published articles or reported experiences in clinical settings to calculate the savings potential for health systems choosing to introduce non-traditional BH services into their CINs/ACOs, it becomes apparent that savings for medical health systems can far exceed the cost of the personnel providing improved BH services, perhaps even signficantly.

Some targeted areas are easier to predict cost savings than others. For instance, introduction of collaborative care into medical outpatient clinics can be expected to reduce total cost of care for program participants by 5% to 15%. While these savings typically do not appear in the first year of the program since this is the health stabilization period, savings that run in the millions of dollars for populations as small as 100,000 have been documented to accrue for up to five years after program participation.

Real savings are also easily documented when psychiatrist-led teams of BH professionals become members of general medical hospitalist teams and assist with concurrent treatment of BH disorder from day one of general hospital admission. This is associated with shorter hospital stays of 0.9 to 3 days and a net return on investment in hospitals with very high censuses and/or a high percentage of at-risk payor arrangements (e.g., DRGs). As a result, general hospital early adopters nationally are subsidizing proactive BH consulation as a means of reducing total health costs, enhancing the quality of care, and improving hospital bottom lines for comorbid medical admissions when these patients are uninsured, underinsured, or insured on a fee per case basis.

During comprehensive evaluations of health systems encompassing 2 to more than 10 hospitals and often hundreds of corresponding medical clinics, it has been possible to estimate millions in annual net savings in a world of population risk-based contracting. The projected savings often allow inclusion/expansion of BH services even when available data is insufficiently developed to support BH service introduction on the basis of actual hospital system analytics (e.g., pediatric and child BH programs).

Doing nothing will predictably be associated with high costs of unnecessary care and declining fee-for-service bases, an unacceptable scenario for systems wishing to increase market share in the future. Thus, informed systems recognize this shortfall as an area of opportunity for improving health and cost management. They grapple with the decision of buying or building a solution. In today's world, buying is really not an option since few, if any, BH organizations deliver BH services effectively in the medical setting. Therefore, several health systems are now in the process of building non-traditional value-added services because they have run their own numbers.

Conclusions

When health systems are developing CINs/ACOs, little thought is given to the inclusion of BH services as a part of core CIN/ACO provider participation and service delivery. For those who do consider BH inclusion, siloed BH payment and independent service delivery procedures quickly drive decision-making leadership to exclude active BH participation due to the logistical challenges.

In this Chapter we make the case that BH comorbidity in the medical setting is associated with medical treatment resistance, especially in complex high cost patients, and large increases in total health care spending, especially for medical services in patients with comorbid BH conditions. Since the primary goal of CINs/ACOs is to improve health and decrease cost, without the inclusion of BH professionals and services as core members and activities in ACOs and many focused CINs, FTC and DOJ requirements will not be met. This is particularly true when one considers that there are now models of non-traditional integrated medical and BH care delivery that predicably attenuate the health and cost consequences of BH conditions in medical settings.

This Chapter recognizes that the inclusion of BH professionals and services in CINs/ACOs creates several challenges for those that are developing them. Therefore, it provides a roadmap that will allow those willing to maximize the effectiveness of their CIN/ACO to achive the Triple Aim.(Berwick, Nolan, & Whittington, 2008)

Chapter 11 Study Questions

Study questions are provided for team building or class exercises. Answers for all questions are provided in Appendix C.

Question Number	Question
1	The expected total cost of care for patients with a chronic illness and a concurrent behavioral health condition compared to a general population of medical patients will be: a. About the same b. Twice as much c. Three to four times as much d. Five to six times as much
2	The majority of increased cost of care for patients with behavioral health conditions is for: a. Medical treatment b. Psychiatric hospitalization c. Psychotropic medication d. Residential care
3	"Carve-out" and "carve-in" managed behavioral health organizations: a. Are owned by the medical insurer that covers medical benefit payments. b. Use payment practices that encourage delivery of behavioral health services in the medical setting. c. Manage networks of behavioral health providers separate and apart from medical providers. d. Use the same claims adjudication procedures as for medical benefits.
4	CINs/ACOs in which behavioral health providers are contracted professional resources but not network members can be expected to: a. Provide easily accessible behavioral health services for high cost, complex network patients. b. Improve clinical outcomes and lower cost in the majority of network patients with behavioral health

Question Number	Question
	comorbidity.
	c. Follow CIN/ACO policies and procedures (referral use, documentation, formularies, clinical guidelines) just as medical specialty network providers.
	d. None of the above
5	What percentage of patients with behavioral health conditions is seen and receives the majority of their BH treatment in the behavioral health sector?

a. 10-20%
b. 30-50%
c. 60-80%
d. 90-100%

6.   On average, the length of stay for medical/surgical inpatients with behavioral health comorbidity is:

a. 1 day shorter due to psychiatric hospital transfer
b. The same
c. 1 day longer
d. 4 days longer

7.   On average, the thirty-day readmission rate for medical/surgical inpatient discharges with behavioral health comorbidity is:

a. >30% higher than those without
b. 20%-30% higher than those without
c. 10%-20% higher than those without
d. 5%-10% higher than those without

Answers to Chapter 11 Study Questions

1. Answer C. Three to four times as much.

2. Answer A. Medical treatment.

3. Answer C. Manage networks of behavioral health providers separate and apart from medical providers.

4. Answer D. None of the above.

5. Answer A. 10-20%

6. Answer C. 1 day longer.

7. Answer A. >30% higher than those without

Chapter 11 Highlights

- Eighty percent of patients with BH conditions are seen in the medical sector.

- BH comorbidity in general medical patients is common, especially in complex high cost patients.

- Untreated, poorly treated BH conditions in general medical patients doubles medical service use and result in a spend four times greater than the spend on BH care.

- The siloed medical and BH payment systems obviates the opportunities for interdisciplinary care coordination and delivery of effective, efficient integrated care.

- Studies of value-added models of integrated medical and BH services delivery demonstrate health improvement, patient satisfaction, and cost reduction.

- CINs without BH network providers delivering BH services in the general medical setting can expect ongoing treatment resistance and high health care costs in comorbid general medical and BH patients.

CHAPTER 11 REFERENCES

Akunne, A., Murthy, L., & Young, J. (2012). Cost-effectiveness of multi-component interventions to prevent delirium in older people admitted to medical wards. *Age Ageing, 41*(3), 285-291. doi: 10.1093/ageing/afr147

Barnett, K., Mercer, S. W., Norbury, M., Watt, G., Wyke, S., & Guthrie, B. (2012). Epidemiology of multimorbidity and implications for health care, research, and medical education: a cross-sectional study. *Lancet, 380*(9836), 37-43. doi: 10.1016/S0140-6736(12)60240-2

Berwick, D. M., Nolan, T. W., & Whittington, J. (2008). The triple aim: care, health, and cost. *Health affairs, 27*(3), 759-769. doi: 10.1377/hlthaff.27.3.759

Bower, P., Knowles, S., Coventry, P. A., & Rowland, N. (2011). Counselling for mental health and psychosocial problems in primary care. *Cochrane database of systematic reviews*(9), CD001025. doi: 10.1002/14651858.CD001025.pub3

Bower, P., Rowland, N., & Hardy, R. (2003). The clinical effectiveness of counselling in primary care: a systematic review and meta-analysis. *Psychological medicine, 33*(02), 203-215.

Chang, C. K., Hayes, R. D., Perera, G., Broadbent, M. T., Fernandes, A. C., Lee, W. E., . . . Stewart, R. (2011). Life expectancy at birth for people with serious mental illness and other major disorders from a secondary mental health care case register in London. *PloS one, 6*(5), e19590. doi: 10.1371/journal.pone.0019590

Chen, C. C., Lin, M. T., Tien, Y. W., Yen, C. J., Huang, G. H., & Inouye, S. K. (2011). Modified hospital elder life program: effects on abdominal surgery patients. *J Am Coll Surg, 213*(2), 245-252. doi: 10.1016/j.jamcollsurg.2011.05.004

Cunningham, P. J. (2009). Beyond parity: primary care physicians' perspectives on access to mental health care. *Health Aff (Millwood), 28*(3), w490-501. doi: hlthaff.28.3.w490 [pii]

10.1377/hlthaff.28.3.w490

Desan, P. H., Zimbrean, P. C., Weinstein, A. J., Bozzo, J. E., & Sledge, W. H. (2011). Proactive psychiatric consultation services reduce length of stay for admissions to an inpatient medical team. *Psychosomatics, 52*(6), 513-520. doi: 10.1016/j.psym.2011.06.002

Druss, B. G., & Walker, E. R. (2011). Mental disorders and medical comorbidity. *The Synthesis project. Research synthesis report*(21), 1-26.

Druss, B. G., Zhao, L., Von Esenwein, S., Morrato, E. H., & Marcus, S. C. (2011). Understanding excess mortality in persons with mental illness: 17-year follow up of a nationally representative US survey. *Med Care, 49*(6), 599-604. doi: 10.1097/MLR.0b013e31820bf86e

Franz, C. E., Barker, J. C., Kim, K., Flores, Y., Jenkins, C., Kravitz, R. L., & Hinton, L. (2010). When help becomes a hindrance: mental health referral systems as barriers to care for primary care physicians treating patients with Alzheimer's disease. *Am J Geriatr Psychiatry, 18*(7), 576-585.

Inouye, S. K., Bogardus, S. T., Jr., Williams, C. S., Leo-Summers, L., & Agostini, J. V. (2003). The role of adherence on the effectiveness of nonpharmacologic interventions: evidence from the delirium prevention trial. *Arch Intern Med, 163*(8), 958-964.

Kathol, R., Lattimer, C., Gold, W., Perez, R., & Gutteridge, D. (2011). Creating clinical and economic "wins" through integrated case management. Lessons for physicians and health system administrators. *Journal of Ambulatory Care Management, 34*(2), 140-151.

Kathol, R., McAlpine, D., Kishi, Y., Spies, R., Meller, W., Bernhardt, T., . . . Gold, W. (2005). General Medical and Pharmacy Claims Expenditures in Users of Behavioral Health Services. *Journal of General Internal Medicine, 20*(2), 160-167.

Kathol, R., Perez, R., & Cohen, J. (2010). *The Integrated Case Management Manual: Assisting Complex Patients Regain Physical and Mental Health* (1st ed.). New York City: Springer Publishing.

Kathol, R. G., deGruy, F., & Rollman, B. L. (in press). Value-Based Financially Sustainable Behavioral Health Components for Patient-Centered Medical Homes. *Ann Fam Med.*

Kathol, R. G., Kunkel, E. J., Weiner, J. S., McCarron, R. M., Worley, L. L., Yates, W. R., . . . Huyse, F. J. (2009). Psychiatrists for the Medically Complex: Bringing Value at the Physical Health & Mental Health Substance Use Disorder Interface. *Psychosomatics, 50*(March-April), 93-107.

Katon, W., Russo, J., Lin, E. H., Schmittdiel, J., Ciechanowski, P., Ludman, E., . . . Von Korff, M. (2012). Cost-effectiveness of a multicondition collaborative care intervention: a randomized controlled trial.

Arch Gen Psychiatry, 69(5), 506-514. doi: 10.1001/archgenpsychiatry.2011.1548

Katon, W. J., Lin, E. H., Von Korff, M., Ciechanowski, P., Ludman, E. J., Young, B., . . . McCulloch, D. (2010). Collaborative care for patients with depression and chronic illnesses. *N Engl J Med, 363*(27), 2611-2620.

Katon, W. J., & Seelig, M. (2008). Population-based care of depression: team care approaches to improving outcomes. *J Occup Environ Med, 50*(4), 459-467.

Kessler, R. C., Demler, O., Frank, R. G., Olfson, M., Pincus, H. A., Walters, E. E., . . . Zaslavsky, A. M. (2005). Prevalence and treatment of mental disorders, 1990 to 2003. *N Engl J Med, 352*(24), 2515-2523.

Larkin, G. L., Claassen, C. A., Emond, J. A., Pelletier, A. J., & Camargo, C. A. (2005). Trends in U.S. emergency department visits for mental health conditions, 1992 to 2001. *Psychiatr Serv., 56*(6), 671-677.

Little-Upah, P., Carson, C., Williamson, R., Williams, T., Cimino, M., Mehta, N., . . . Kisiel, S. (2013). The Banner psychiatric center: a model for providing psychiatric crisis care to the community while easing behavioral health holds in emergency departments. *Perm J, 17*(1), 45-49. doi: 10.7812/TPP/12-016

Lucas, R., Farley, H., Twanmoh, J., Urumov, A., Evans, B., & Olsen, N. (2009). Measuring the opportunity loss of time spent boarding admitted patients in the emergency department: a multihospital analysis. *J Healthc Manag, 54*(2), 117-124; discussion 124-115.

Manderscheid, R., & Kathol, R. G. (in press). Fostering Sustainable, Integrated Medical and Behavioral Health Services in Medical Settings. *AIM*.

Melek, S., Norris, D. T., & Paulus, J. (2013). Economic Impact of Integrated Medical-Behavioral Healthcare: Implications for Psychiatry. In A. P. Press (Ed.). Arlington VA: American Psychiatric Assoication.

Ostbye, T., Yarnall, K. S., Krause, K. M., Pollak, K. I., Gradison, M., & Michener, J. L. (2005). Is there time for management of patients with chronic diseases in primary care? *Annals of family medicine, 3*(3), 209-214. doi: 10.1370/afm.310

Pratt, R., MacGregor, A., Reid, S., & Given, L. (2012). Wellness Recovery Action Planning (WRAP) in self-help and mutual support groups. *Psychiatr Rehabil J, 35*(5), 403-405. doi: 10.1037/h0094501

Prince, M., Patel, V., Saxena, S., Maj, M., Maselko, J., Phillips, M. R., & Rahman, A. (2007). No health without mental health. *Lancet, 370*(9590), 859-877. doi: S0140-6736(07)61238-0 [pii]

10.1016/S0140-6736(07)61238-0

Regier, D. A., Narrow, W. E., Rae, D. S., Manderscheid, R. W., Locke, B. Z., & Goodwin, F. K. (1993). The de facto US mental and addictive disorders service system. Epidemiologic catchment area prospective 1-year prevalence rates of disorders and services. *Arch Gen Psychiatry, 50*(2), 85-94.

Reilly, S., Planner, C., Hann, M., Reeves, D., Nazareth, I., & Lester, H. (2012). The role of primary care in service provision for people with severe mental illness in the United Kingdom. *PloS one, 7*(5), e36468. doi: 10.1371/journal.pone.0036468

Richmond, T. S., Hollander, J. E., Ackerson, T. H., Robinson, K., Gracias, V., Shults, J., & Amsterdam, J. (2007). Psychiatric disorders in patients presenting to the Emergency Department for minor injury. *Nurs Res, 56*(4), 275-282. doi: 10.1097/01.NNR.0000280616.13566.84

Seelig, M. D., & Katon, W. (2008). Gaps in depression care: why primary care physicians should hone their depression screening, diagnosis, and management skills. *J Occup Environ Med, 50*(4), 451-458.

U.S. Department of Justice, & Federal Trade Commission. (1996). Statements of Antitrust Enforcement Policy in Health Care. . from http://www.justice.gov/atr/public/guidelines/0000.htm

Unutzer, J., Chan, Y. F., Hafer, E., Knaster, J., Shields, A., Powers, D., & Veith, R. C. (2012). Quality improvement with pay-for-performance incentives in integrated behavioral health care. *Am J Public Health, 102*(6), e41-45. doi: 10.2105/AJPH.2011.300555

Unutzer, J., Katon, W. J., Fan, M. Y., Schoenbaum, M. C., Lin, E. H., Della Penna, R. D., & Powers, D. (2008). Long-term cost effects of collaborative care for late-life depression. *Am J Manag Care, 14*(2), 95-100. doi: 7019 [pii]

Wang, P. S., Aguilar-Gaxiola, S., Alonso, J., Angermeyer, M. C., Borges, G., Bromet, E. J., . . . Wells, J. E. (2007). Use of mental health services for anxiety, mood, and substance disorders in 17 countries in the WHO world mental health surveys. *Lancet, 370*(9590), 841-850. doi: 10.1016/S0140-6736(07)61414-7

Wang, P. S., Berglund, P., Olfson, M., Pincus, H. A., Wells, K. B., & Kessler, R. C. (2005). Failure and delay in initial treatment contact after first onset of mental disorders in the National Comorbidity Survey Replication. *Arch Gen Psychiatry, 62*(6), 603-613.

Wang, P. S., Demler, O., & Kessler, R. C. (2002). Adequacy of treatment for serious mental illness in the United States. *Am J Public Health, 92*(1), 92-98.

Wang, P. S., Demler, O., Olfson, M., Pincus, H. A., Wells, K. B., & Kessler, R. C. (2006). Changing profiles of service sectors used for mental health care in the United States. *Am J Psychiatry, 163*(7), 1187-1198. doi: 10.1176/appi.ajp.163.7.1187

Wang, P. S., Lane, M., Olfson, M., Pincus, H. A., Wells, K. B., & Kessler, R. C. (2005). Twelve-month use of mental health services in the United States: results from the National Comorbidity Survey Replication. *Arch Gen Psychiatry, 62*(6), 629-640.

Wang, W., Li, H. L., Wang, D. X., Zhu, X., Li, S. L., Yao, G. Q., . . . Zhu, S. N. (2012). Haloperidol prophylaxis decreases delirium incidence in elderly patients after noncardiac surgery: a randomized controlled trial*. *Crit Care Med, 40*(3), 731-739. doi: 10.1097/CCM.0b013e3182376e4f

Woltmann, E., Grogan-Kaylor, A., Perron, B., Georges, H., Kilbourne, A. M., & Bauer, M. S. (2012). Comparative effectiveness of collaborative chronic care models for mental health conditions across primary, specialty, and behavioral health care settings: systematic review and meta-analysis. *Am J Psychiatry, 169*(8), 790-804. doi: 10.1176/appi.ajp.2012.11111616

Yarnall, K. S., Pollak, K. I., Ostbye, T., Krause, K. M., & Michener, J. L. (2003). Primary care: is there enough time for prevention? *Am J Public Health, 93*(4), 635-641.

www.ingramcontent.com/pod-product-compliance
Lightning Source LLC
Chambersburg PA
CBHW062029210326
41519CB00060B/7370